"Teens will be sharing this book with their friends everywhere! It's a must read for young people who want to feel good, be smart, and make positive change"

Sophee McPhee, Editor - UP! Magazine

"A realistic look at an unrealistic world. Educating youth on these matters can only lead to improved self-esteem in adulthood"

Renee Kelly, Childhood Psychologist

Does my bum look big in this ad? Lisa Cox
Published by Wombat Books
P. O. Box 1519, Capalaba Qld 4157, Australia
www.wombatbooks.com.au

978-1-921633-05-8

Copyright © Lisa Cox, 2010
www.lisacoxpresents.com

Cover Illustration: Amanda Dunne
Book Illustrations: Amanda Dunne

Printed in Thailand by Thai Watana Panich Press Co, Ltd

National Library of Australia Cataloguing-in-Publication entry
Author: Cox, Lisa.
Title: Does my bum look big in this ad? : body image and the media / Lisa Cox ; illustrator, Amanda Dunne.
Edition: 1st ed.
ISBN: 9781921633058 (pbk.)
Target Audience: For secondary school age.
Subjects: Media literacy--Juvenile literature.
Other Authors/Contributors:
Dunne, Amanda.
Dewey Number: 302.230835

All rights reserved. No part of this publication may be reproduced, stored in, or introduced into a retrieval system, or transmitted, in any form, or by any means (electronic, mechanical, photocopying, recording or otherwise) without the prior written permission of the publisher.

Does my bum look big in this ad?

Body image and the media

Lisa Cox

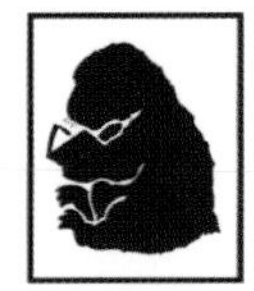

Wombat Books

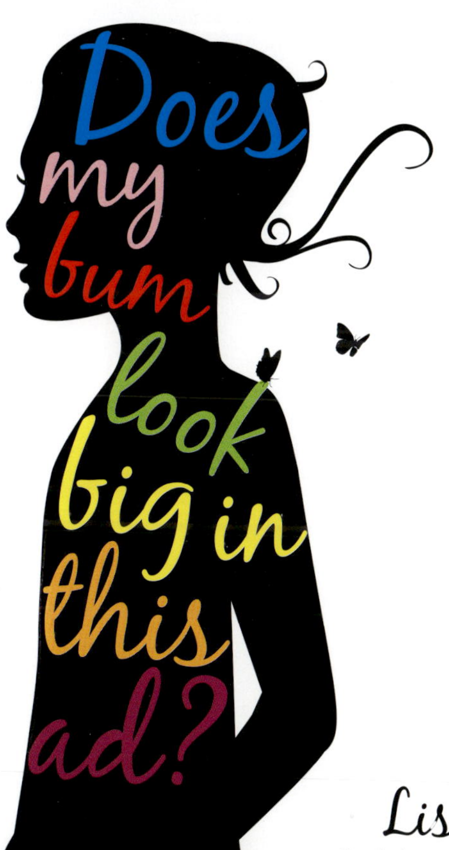

Lisa Cox

Body image and the media

Preface

Ever wondered why you don't look like the people in magazine ads? How does that make you feel?

There are heaps of books about how popular culture, including advertising, affects the way you feel about yourself. Unfortunately, they're mostly written *about* young people… until now!

This book is written *for* young people. We take a behind the scenes look at how the media industry works, teaching you to critically and independently evaluate what you see, hear or read in popular culture, such as the media.

You'll also learn how to develop and maintain a positive body image as you navigate your way through the media maze.

It's time to take control of your body image, instead of having it controlled by others!

Contents

Foreword

For parents and educators

Squeezed in bookshelves and websites around the world is a bulging body of literature describing the effects of popular culture on body image. These books, reports, and articles all discuss, in accurate detail, the damaging and distorting consequences that unrealistic images have on how our children, our students and how we perceive our own body as well as others. And these images bombard us everyday in popular culture.

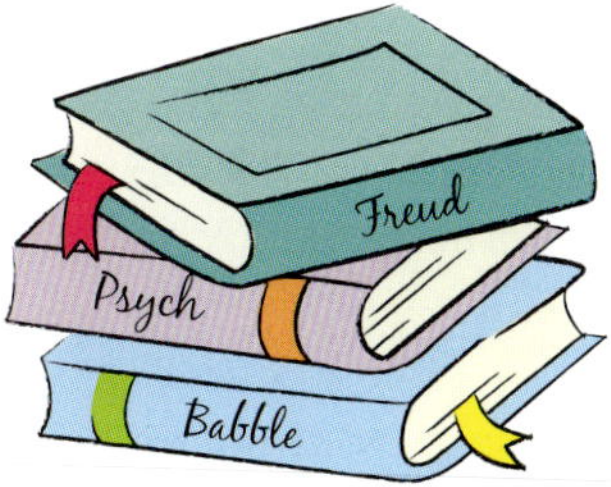

Numerous studies have shown direct correlation between body image perspective and popular culture. For example, the prevalence of underweight models in advertising has been shown to increase the reported incidence of body dissatisfaction, particularly among young people.

You may well wonder why, if there's so much information and so many resources available, there is still such a lack of awareness, understanding and media literacy among our youth? And why do rates of eating disorders continue to rise?

The answer is simple. The vast majority of literature on this topic, to date, is written about young people, not for young people.

Does my bum look big in this ad? is different. With input and contributions from several key professionals in related fields, this book looks objectively at how popular culture impacts young body image - but it is written and presented in a way that a younger audience can understand, appreciate, enjoy and, ultimately, learn from.

You wouldn't want your child to travel into a foreign country without at least a map or phrasebook, would you? But every day, thousands of young people are stepping into the foreign world of popular culture without guidance or even a slight understanding of the manipulating messages they're being exposed to, or what's really going on 'behind the scenes'. Think of this book as a 'guidebook' for navigating through today's hazy media and cultural maze.

Importantly, this book does not aim to dispute other literature on the subject or lay the blame on a particular industry, group, or profession. *Does my bum look big in this ad?* can be used as a fun, informative, educational tool. It aspires to help young people sift through the mixed messages and the barrage of manipulated images they are exposed to. And keep their body image and self-esteem intact.

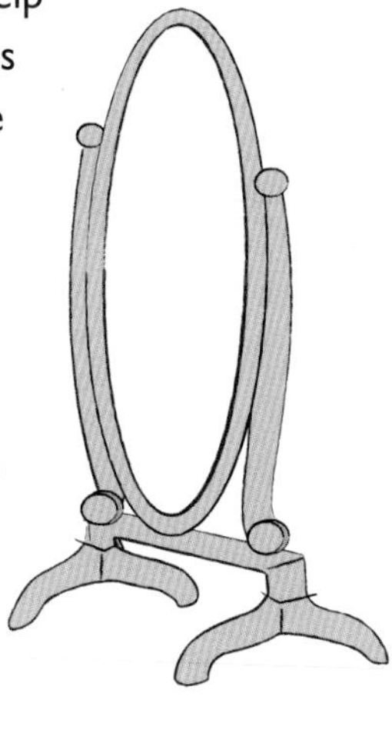

Through simple education and enhanced media literacy, our youth can proactively and independently weed out the superfluous, differentiate fact from fiction and in the end, have the real power of beauty that comes from acceptance, confidence and empowerment.

Body image dissatisfaction is a complex issue with many contributing factors - such as peers, parents, technology and the education system. This book is written for teenagers but you can find more information about the role that you (as a parent, guardian or teacher) can play in the development of a positive, healthy body image at:

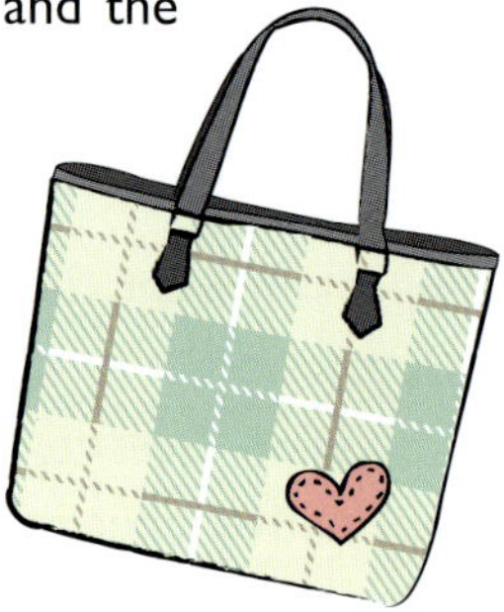

www.MuseInTheMirror.com

Introduction

So what's this book about, anyway?

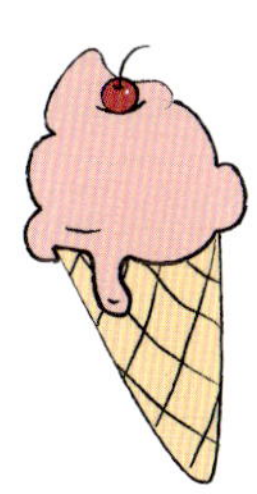

Hi there. We're so glad you're reading this book. So you want to know more about how popular culture affects your body image and the way you feel about YOU? Well, let's start by saying congratulations to you. If knowledge is power, you'll be a very powerful consumer, after reading this book!

There are already heaps of books, articles, and websites out there about popular culture, body image, and other related topics. But... instead of another academic blah-blah book that's just written about you, this one's written for you.

We've tried to leave all the fancy, psycho-babble in the textbooks gathering dust at the back of the library. But if there's a term you just don't get, you can try and Google it (if you haven't already).

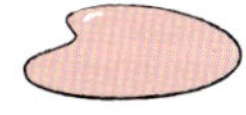

Here's one important thing you should also know... The contents of this book have not been 'dumbed down for youth'. In putting this book together, we've spoken to heaps (thousands, actually) of young people, and one thing they've all agreed on is that they really do want to educate themselves on the topics this book addresses: popular culture, advertising, body image and all that stuff. Except that there were no good books out there to help them do it - until now!

This book will teach you to think critically about how the media and popular culture influence your life and your body image. So the next time you're watching television or reading a magazine, you can make informed and educated decisions for yourself about what you're seeing or hearing. No more feeling bad over those 'perfect' bodies on the magazine covers (which, by the way, probably aren't real, but we'll talk more about that later on in this book). You'll also pick up useful tips for developing and maintaining a positive body image, despite negative influences from things like the media and peer pressure.

Media What?

We want to help you be more ***media literate.*** Media literacy is really just a fancy way of talking about how you interpret and understand all the media you're exposed to. If you were 'computer literate', for example, you'd have a good understanding of computers and be able to use them plus understand the basics of how they work.

Media literacy is also about thinking for yourself, empowering yourself, making decisions for yourself, and realising that YOU ultimately control what is presented in the media. That's right! You control popular culture, and you don't need a Journalism degree to do that. You're in charge – from the swipe of a credit card to the click of a computer mouse or the press of a television remote.

Improving your media literacy can also give you greater appreciation for a diversity of body types – including your own. But right now though, this book is your ultimate must-have accessory for cruising through popular culture. Happy reading!

Chapter One

What's body image and all that stuff?

Well, we should probably start by defining one of the words used a lot throughout this book – body image. But first, here's a pop quiz for you: What do you think about your body after reading a glossy magazine and seeing all the ads in it?

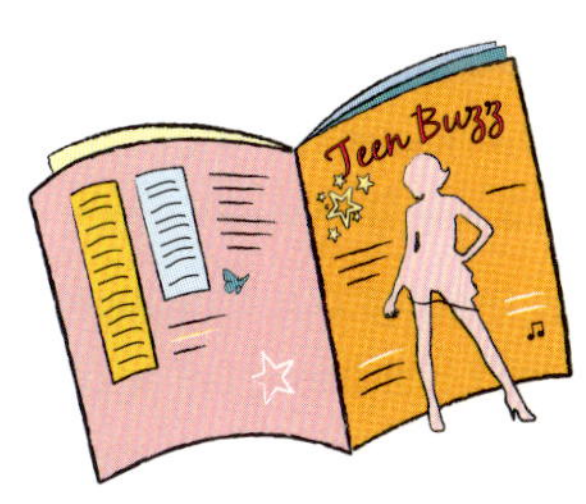

Do you think you're:

a) too fat

b) too skinny

c) too short

d) too tall

e) just right?

If your answer is E, that's great... But, unfortunately, you're a healthy minority. You see, body image is what you think about your own

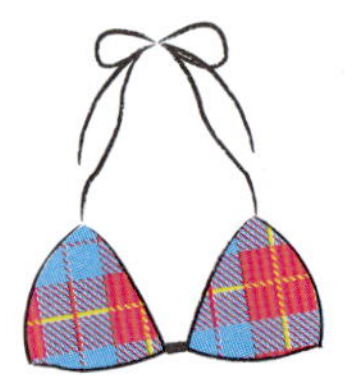

body. It also includes what you think about other bodies and what you think other people are saying about your body.

A positive body image means that you are generally happy with your body shape and size.

A person with a healthy body image takes care of his or her physical and mental health, while respecting themselves and others.

On the other hand, a poor body image (also called body dissatisfaction) means you aren't happy with your body and will focus on the 'bad' aspects, which aren't even bad anyway! You'll read more about developing and maintaining a positive body image throughout this book – especially in Chapter Seven. Poor body image isn't just being unhappy with the painful graze on your knee. It goes much deeper. Comparing your body with the ones you see in advertisements isn't just crazy, it's dangerous and can contribute to the development of serious physical and mental health concerns, such as eating disorders and depression.

Every time you hear or read the news, there seems to be another statistic about how unhappy people are with their body. Depending on which study you read, the statistics change. But one thing that all the body dissatisfaction statistics have in common – they're always high.

So don't feel bad if you don't love your looks every minute of every day. You're certainly not the only person feeling this way – but you are the only person who can make the choices necessary to change the way you feel about yourself!

Remember that things like your genetic makeup play an extremely important role in what you look like. Some people are tall, some are short, some have round faces where others have oval-shaped faces, some people are blonde where others are redheads. These differences are what make you wonderfully unique. You don't need to change them.

We don't all grow at the same rate either. It's just normal that some people go through growth spurts before others. Fact: an 8 year-old will never have the body of an 18 year-old. Keep reminding yourself that it's less important if you grow taller before or after your friends. What matters more is that you're happy and healthy! Chapter Six also looks at factors influencing your body image.

Kids and kilos

The age range of boys and girls with body dissatisfaction also seems to be slippery-dipping down at an alarming rate. Media reports have confirmed that children (that's right: children) as young as six years old are now being hospitalised with eating disorders and dreaming of the day they can have breast implants, like their 'beautiful' role models in the media.

The fairytale diet

We've probably all been on the fairytale diet at some stage – even without realising it. Little kids might not have their body image shaped primarily by glossy magazines and music film clips. Instead, it's the princess's perfectly proportioned body, the chiselled features of handsome prince charmings and dolls with flawless skin or full breasts that influence (and distort) our perceptions of a realistic, ideal body image from a really early age.

Cartoon characters never have obesity problems and dolls never have to worry about pimples. That's because, just like the pictures in the magazines, they're not real! But little kids just aren't equipped with media literacy skills to know the difference. You could say characters like Barbie, Cinderella and Aladdin are supermodels for boys and girls.

The benefits of a positive body image

Just like your body needs you to feed it a healthy diet, your self-esteem needs you to feed it positive, healthy thoughts. Abusing your body with stuff that's bad for it can lead to poor overall health. In a similar way, abusing your mind with negative thoughts can lead to poor mental and physical health.

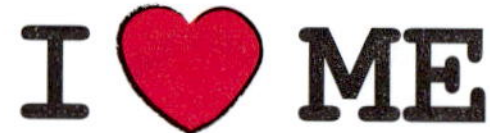

Feeling good about the way you look doesn't make you 'conceited' or 'full-of-yourself'. Feeling good about your body and the way you are is essential.

You're in training

Learning how to overcome challenges is an important part of personal growth, and it promotes a positive self-esteem. If you can't look past your body blues now, how will you learn to overcome the bigger challenges you're bound to face when you get older?

How you look and feel IS important to you but remember that you have much 'bigger' challenges to face later in life: buying a house, raising a family, getting a job or even getting your drivers license. These are challenges you'll want to prepare yourself for (maybe not right now, but eventually). So consider this phase in your life as training for the future.

Learning to accept and appreciate your body at an early age (despite media pressures) will boost your self-esteem and confidence – right now and in coming years as well. Nobody can take that power from you if you don't want them to. That's what a positive body image does for you:

You take charge of your body and your life. You're 100% in control!

Now isn't that the most beautiful and most empowering thing you can do for yourself?

So here's the deal...

Here's what we've established so far: improving your media literacy can have a positive influence on your body image. In turn, a positive body image builds positive self-esteem. The stronger your self-esteem, the less vulnerable you are to negative influences in your life (like bullies and peer pressure and the media).

Let's say you have a poor body image and you're reading a magazine. As you leaf through pages showing a young female with full breasts, a slim waist, really awesome clothes, flawless, glowing skin and shining hair, how do you begin to feel about yourself? Maybe you're scrutinising your own reflection and wondering why you don't look like her?!!!

But wait...

Good media literacy = Positive body image and self-esteem

As you flick through that same magazine you know that, in real life, the girl in the magazine looks nothing like her photo. With a positive body image you won't be comparing your own body against the digitally altered bodies in the magazine.

Here are a few more benefits to having a positive body image:

- Reduced stress, which can be responsible for things like pimples and mood swings.
- Enhanced relationships with your family and friends.
- Improved performance at school and in sports.
- Less chance of being upset by bullies and peer pressure.
- Plus... Stronger appeal to the opposite sex.

Yep, forget the size of your hips or your muscles. A positive, healthy body image is the best-looking accessory you'll ever have. Wohoo!

Body bullies and positive peers

Having a positive body image is one challenge; surrounding yourself with like-minded, positive peers is another. It is critical that you find these empowering friends, who won't deflate your self-esteem. 'Body bullies' make you feel bad about your body with a single comment or glance. No matter what their physical appearance, this behavior makes people *REALLY UGLY*.

You might be surprised to know that these same people (the body bullies) are often the ones lacking self-confidence. Sadly, making nasty comments about your body is one way for them to feel better about themselves. Do you really want people like that around you? The point here is to spend more time with people who make you feel good about you. (Psst... There are more tips on getting a positive body image in Chapter Seven.)

Ban 'fat-talk' today!

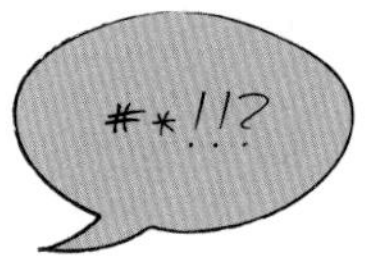

Sitting around with your friends and talking about all the things you hate about your bodies is *NOT OK*. It can make you a body bully without even realising it. So next time your friend complains about something to do with the size or shape of his or her body, remind them of all their great qualities that people admire… including those things that aren't physical – like his or her kind personality.

Homework

- List three things you like about yourself. Remember they don't have to be physical so you can include your great sense of humor or thoughtful personality. Then perhaps you and your friends can do the same for each other too!

Chapter Two

What's up with popular culture?

Let's go back to popular culture for a while. Popular culture (also known as pop culture) is basically the attitudes, ideals, social norms and perspectives in mainstream culture.

When we talk about popular culture in this book, we're mostly referring to Western culture. In this instance, popular culture may include all sorts of things: music, sports, art, fashion, advertising, television shows and movies, just to name a few.

Advertising makes up a massive part of popular culture. Each day, you can expect to be exposed to thousands of ads. It's also estimated that the average adult spends about one and a half years

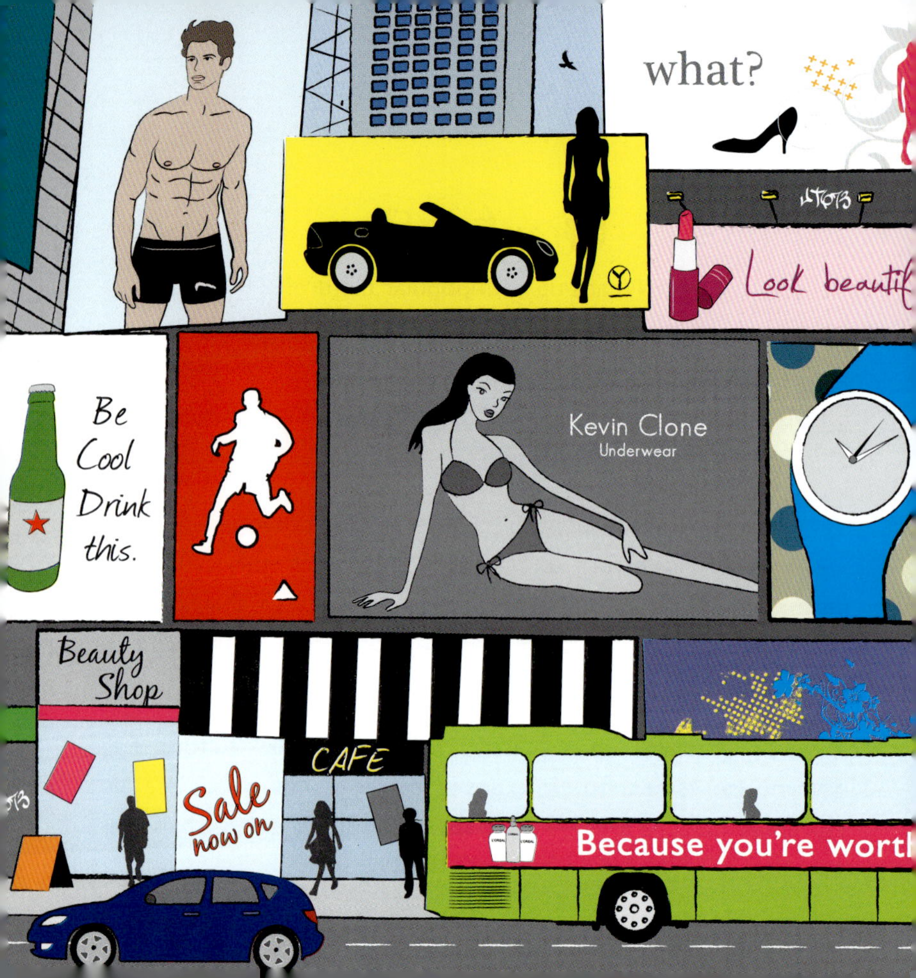

what?
Look beautif
Be
Cool
Drink
this.
Kevin Clone
Underwear
Beauty
Shop
CAFE
Sale
now on
Because you're wortl

of his life viewing or listening to ads. You can only expect this time to increase as we spend less time in the park and more time surfing the internet. That amounts to a lot of outside influence coming at you every day from just *one* element of popular culture.

It's no secret that the advertising world is a massive, multi-billion dollar industry. It's also extremely powerful.

One of the primary purposes of advertising is to reinforce the value society places on things like physical beauty.

No matter how much you may *think* it doesn't affect you, it does. From the day you were born and your parents drove you home from the hospital in a Honda, dressed you in Bonds, and used Huggies wet wipes to change your K-mart nappy, advertising has played a role in your life - whether you realise it or not and whether you like it or not.

Just like this very moment. You might be reading an e-book on your Toshiba laptop, listening to your iPod, waiting for a call on your Nokia phone, and tugging at the loose threads of your Target socks. It's virtually impossible not to be influenced by advertising.

A brief history of advertising

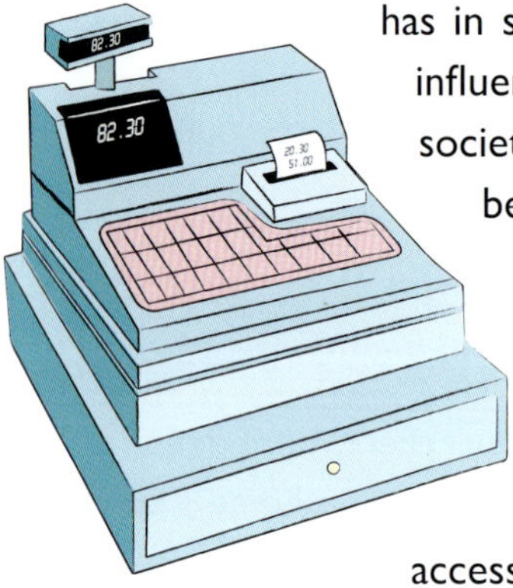

We can't underestimate the immense power advertising has in shaping our lives. It's arguably the most influential and educational force in today's society. But it wasn't always like this. You see, before mass media took over our lives, things like religion and family played a much more important role in shaping the lives of the generations before us. Now, as technology advances and with information accessible with a click of the mouse, popular culture has invaded your home, your time, your body, and your life. Teens in the 1800's didn't watch video clips on their mobile phones while at the bus stop, did they?

Is all advertising going to ruin my body image?

No. Not all advertising is manipulative and deceitful. In fact, some advertising can actually be helpful. For example, if an advertisment is promoting a discount at the grocery store, this might help you save money. You might choose Product A instead of Product B because the advertisements told you that Product A is cheaper. This is not sneaky, manipulative advertising that distorts our body image.

But what if you bought Product A in the hope it will give you a body like the model in the ad? Or what if you bought Product A because you thought it would make you more popular?

Advertising can be helpful but it can also be harmful by affecting the way you feel about yourself.

That's why improving your media literacy is so important.

Knowing how to independently interpret the different messages that you see, hear or read in popular culture is key to developing and maintaining a positive, healthy body image.

Homework

- Find advertisements in a magazine that make you feel good about your own body and promote a positive body image. Now, find advertisements that do the opposite and leave you feeling bad about your own appearance.
- Why do you think the advertisers did this?
- How would you change the advertisement? The words in the headline? Maybe the model or what he/she is wearing?
- You might also want to talk about this with a parent or friend. They may even think the same way you do!

But aren't there codes of conduct?

Governments and organisations around the world have tried (and sometimes succeeded) for years to alter what advertisers can say and how they can say it. But often, these codes are not obligatory and not particularly influential. As you'll read later on, the real powers of influence begin with you.

Air-shop, Photo-brush etc...

You might have read about or heard of terms like airbrushing, retouching, Photoshop and digital enhancement – in this book or in the media. These words are all very similar and relate to how images are altered on a computer before they appear in popular culture.

For example, a photograph of a female body can be digitally enhanced on the computer by using the airbrush tool to make pimples disappear or make breasts bigger and a waistline smaller.

We won't go into too much detail describing the computer software or hardware. Plus, with technology changing so quickly, there could be new applications on the market before you finish reading this book! Unless you're becoming a professional retoucher, you don't need an intimate understanding of all the complicated computer talk.

Chapter Three

Boys, botox and boobs

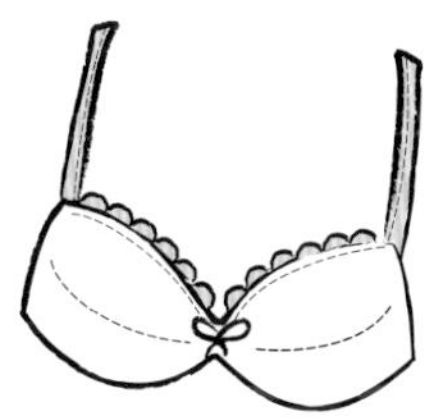

According to your average advertisement in most women's magazines, we could all probably lose a few kilos, have our teeth straighter and whiter, skin that's acne-free, thighs firmer, legs longer, stomach toned… oh and larger, perky breasts would make you a better person, of course!

This chapter looks at how women are depicted in advertising. But listen up, boys and men: this chapter is still relevant to you, so don't flick to the next chapter just yet. In the same way that advertising can dictate how females should look and behave, it also dictates how males should expect a girl – a friend, girlfriend, sister, or even a mother - to look and behave. Real people (male or female) don't really look like the people in the magazines. When you read on, you'll see that a lot of professionals work together to 'perfect' the person you see in the ad or the magazine.

You should also know that when the word 'women' or 'woman' is used here, it also includes younger teenage and pre-teen girls (or vice-versa). Similarly, you can often substitute 'woman' for 'man' and the core message remains. Just as airbrushed breasts create an unrealistic body image for girls and women, airbrushed muscles create equally unrealistic body images for boys and men.

Plus, in the same way pimples are airbrushed on teenagers, wrinkles are airbrushed on older people too.

The Lipstick Revolution: Women in popular culture

Let's continue this journey through the media maze by looking at the changes that have shaped the landscape of popular Western culture. Issues surrounding the misrepresentation of women in popular culture have been around for years. But social, cultural, and industrial changes over the years have altered how women are depicted in advertising.

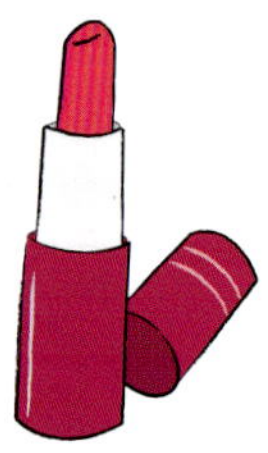

Women today have a higher percentage of spending power compared to previous generations. If you're a teen today, you might think it's normal for males and females to have equal rights in school and in the workplace. But this wasn't always the case.

Consequently, advertisers have mirrored this trend. In order to have a better grasp of the female market, advertisers have revised the ways in which women are represented in advertising. For example, advertisers once made car ads solely targeted at men. These days, it is more common for that family car advertisement to be aimed at females and address their needs and desires.

While there is nothing wrong about women becoming the target market of advertising, what is wrong is *how* women have been used (or misused) in advertising. Their bodies, particularly, have become the primary platforms for many advertising campaigns. You may have seen men and women airbrushed to perfection just to sell toothpaste. Where's the credibility in that?

Role models in popular culture

With more and more women entering popular culture (a really good thing, by the way), increasing numbers of women are being crowned as 'role models'. But sadly, many of these people don't realise the honour that has been bestowed on them.

So why were they called role models to begin with? Was it because of their bra size or their ability to fit into super-skinny jeans?

It seems we've become so obsessed with physical appearances, that we've come to associate them with greatness.

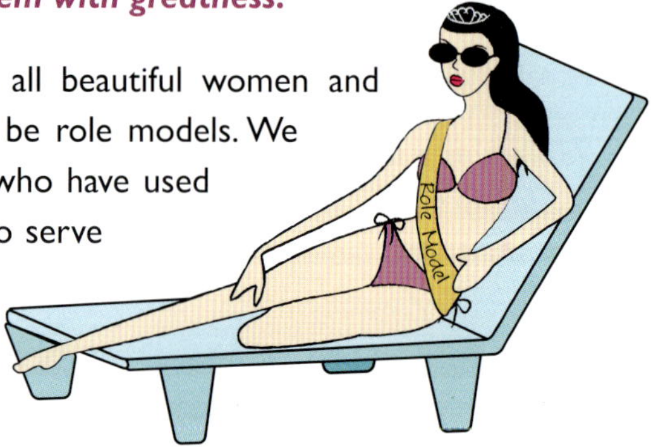

This is not to say that all beautiful women and men do not deserve to be role models. We can name some people who have used their beauty and talent to serve worthy causes. What we're merely saying is this: let us not be so quick to crown anyone with the 'role model' title just because he/she is rich, physically beautiful or famous. Let us choose wisely the people who will inspire and motivate us.

Or better yet, be your own motivation and inspiration. It is your life. You know best how to live it. Your best role model isn't the person in the magazine… it's the person smiling back at you in the mirror.

Homework

- List your biggest role models. Then think about why you look up to them.

Chapter Four

Media smoke and mirrors

The media is guilty of contradicting itself on issues relating to body image by saying or publishing messages that are polar-opposites.

For example, you might have seen magazine covers with bold headlines that say things like 'Love your body,' but on the next page you see an ultra-slim or ultra-muscular, airbrushed model that makes you feel bad about your own appearance.

Or perhaps you've noticed media reports ridiculing models who are 'too thin'. Then in the next program, issue or website, healthy-looking celebrities are criticised for their weight gain (which is often just the camera angle anyway!).

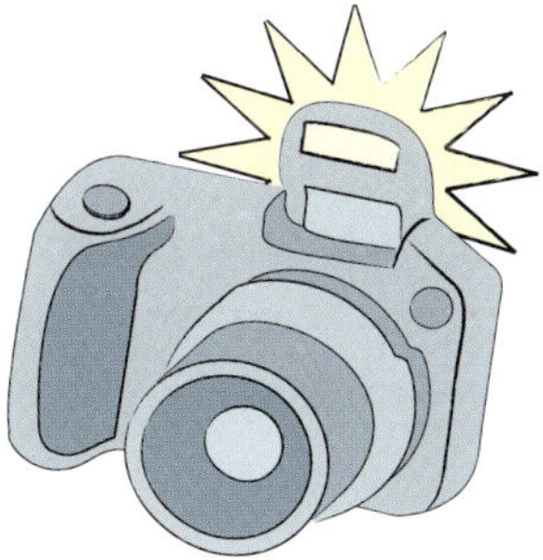

This is a complete contradiction and being aware that this happens – and not letting it upset you – is all a part of being media literate.

How the media operates

Mass media - TV, radio, and print - is there, primarily, to inform and entertain us. However, it is also run like a business. It has staffing costs, other overheads and revenue. So, all the bigwigs in the media industry think like business people, of course, and aim to make a profit.

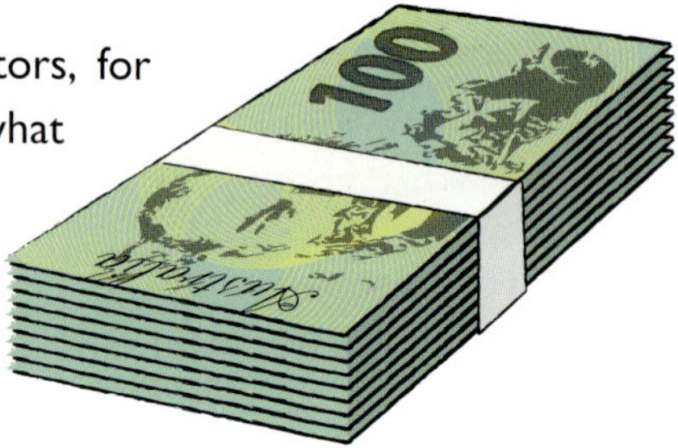

Most (but not all) magazine editors, for example, base their content on what sells. So going by the current popular culture out there, things like sex, celebrity, glamour and gossip sell like crazy! That's why the media pushes things like 'latest celebrity diet tips' – it sells.

This doesn't mean it's right, but it is reality.

People in popular culture related industries don't live with their head in the sand. They are well aware of the power they have to shape your attitudes, values and beliefs.

Popular culture wittingly or unwittingly, sends out the wrong message about how you should look and feel. But as your media literacy improves, you won't be misled by messages that have a negative impact on your body image.

Inspiring insecurity

Often, advertisers will try to make their brand inspirational to you, the consumer. But, ironically, they'll use unattainable and unrealistic images to do this in their ads – which just leaves you feeling like rubbish with a damaged self-esteem.

What's inspirational about that?!

Picture not-so-perfect

Trust us, when a model walks in to be photographed, they hardly resemble the 'finished product' you see in the ad. But most of us might already know that. So let's clear up a few more advertising and media myths.

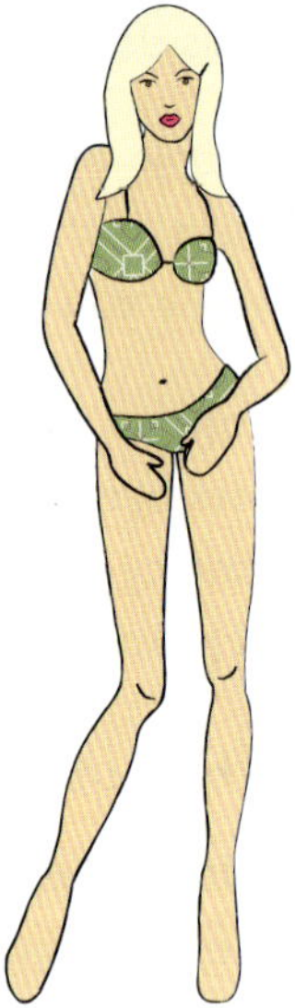

Myth - all airbrushing is bad

Airbrushing, digital enhancement and retouching (they're basically the same thing as we already mentioned) are frequently misused and misunderstood terms.

The truth is, in advertisements, nearly ***everything*** is airbrushed. From the apples in the grocery catalogue to the houses in the real estate brochure, chances are that the image has been digitally altered in some way. But this isn't the problem. An airbrushed car tyre, for example, doesn't leave you feeling unattractive and worthless. This is the problem - when the airbrushed images manipulate and distort our perceptions of what our body should look like. It's a problem when the altered images are passed off as how a 'normal' body should look. A model can lose weight or gain bigger muscles with a few clicks of the computer mouse.

Psst... There are a heap of video examples online if you want to check them out – **www.MuseInTheMirror.com** has a few of our favorites.

Homework

- You don't have to write anything this time. Just look around you at popular culture - which builds your awareness and media literacy.
- Take a closer look at ALL advertising – even in the grocery catalogue. Notice how the fruit and vegetables are always 'perfect' (without bruises and blemishes).
- Look out for 'contradictions' in the media (like we mentioned above). You might want to talk about them with others.

Chapter Five

Behind the scenes at a photo shoot

So you're wondering why the photo you took last weekend of you and your friends doesn't look anything like the people in the magazines? Let us take you behind the scenes on any given photo shoot for an advertisement or magazine article. A typical shoot is created by a team of at least eight people:

1. a Photographer,
2. at least one Lighting Assistant,
3. a Makeup Artist,
4. a Hairstylist,
5. an Art Director,
6. a Stylist,
7. a Stylist's Assistant,
8. and the Model, of course.

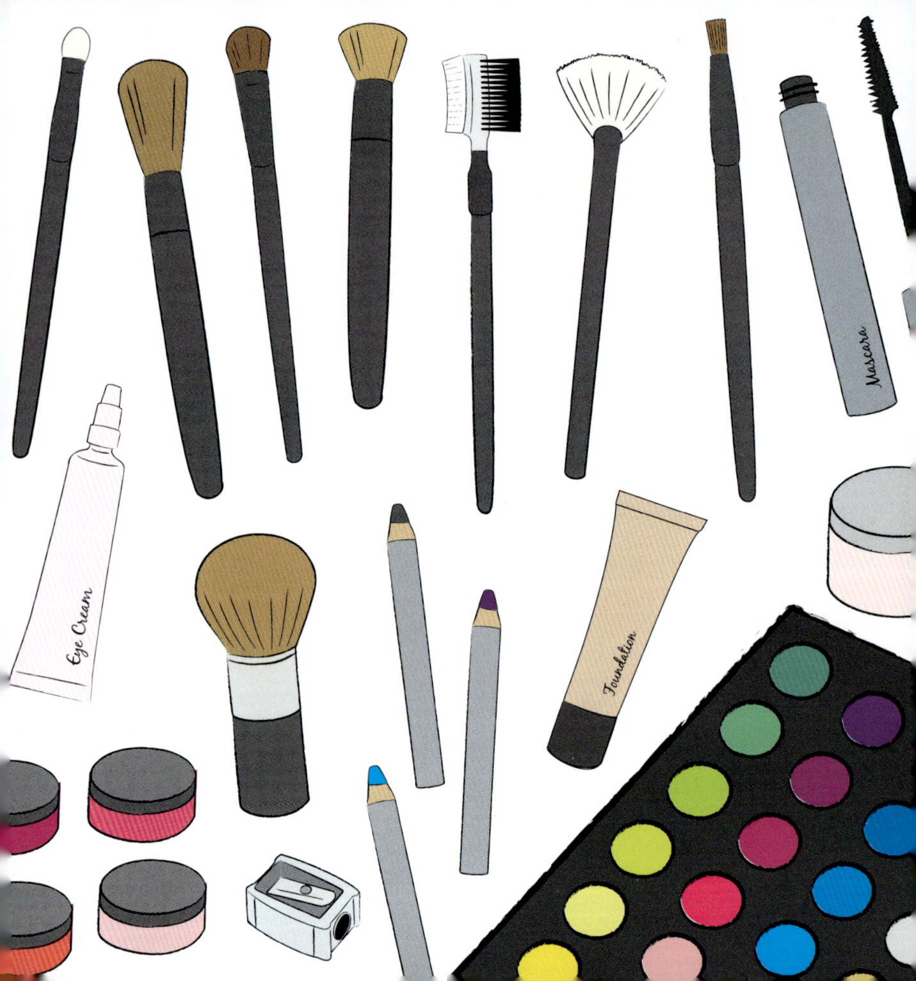
Mascara
Eye Cream
Foundation

They all work together to create and capture the right shot.

The Makeup Artist goes to work, covering blemishes, putting on false eyelashes while the Hairstylist may use hair extensions. The Stylist directs the whole look and puts together the most stylish, slimming outfits. You wouldn't recognise the model as the makeup-free person who wore a casual tracksuit an hour before!

Then... the Photographer tests lights and camera angles. The wrong angles make the model look older, paler, shorter or bigger. Hundreds of photos are taken, but only one is chosen.

Even the 'airbrush-free' images in the media still have LOTS of help to achieve flawless perfection. Before an image is retouched, things like makeup, styling, camera angles and lighting (as we just mentioned) can alter our perceptions of reality - all before the computerised post-production even begins!

These days, with the latest technology, it's not just still photos that can be manipulated. Video and film can also go through a similar post-production process.

The wonders of Photoshop

Then… the magic begins: welcome to the world of Photoshop where images are airbrushed and retouched beyond belief. Pimples and freckles are erased, waistlines are shrunk, cleavage enhanced, legs lengthened… and so on. A model can barely recognise his or her own body after post-production!

Nothing escapes airbrushing, not even those models who are already stunning to begin with. That's how unrealistic these images are. So let's be realistic.

Real people have flaws. It's okay to have one, or two, or three, or more. Actually, it's not just ok to have flaws...

IT'S NORMAL!

Chapter Six

The blame game

So who is responsible for these misrepresentations, distortions, and manipulations of body image in popular culture? Here are some of the usual guilty suspects:

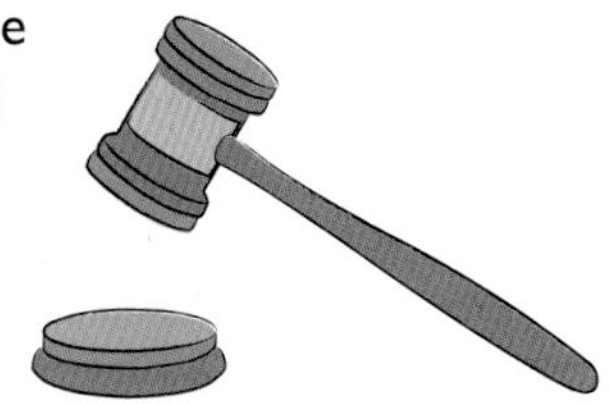

Parents

Have you ever heard your Mum or Dad talk about their wobbly legs, big stomach or wrinkles? Children are like sponges, taking on the positive and negative body image of their parents from a very young age.

Peers and friends

It's not called 'peer pressure' for nothing. You might not realise it but your peers have tremendous influence over your body image. But remember that REAL friends don't judge you for your physical appearance! You can read more about 'body bullies' and 'fat-talk' in Chapter One.

Technology

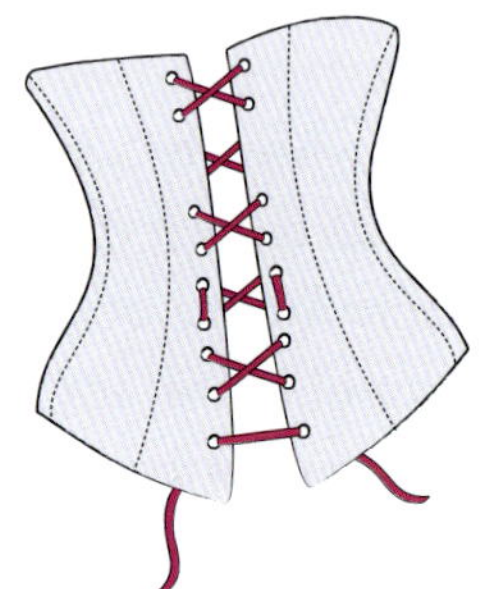

The airbrush is referred to as the 21st century corset and in many ways, it is. You can read about how the airbrush changes images in Chapter Five.

The media

I think we've covered the bases here, haven't we?

BUT… It is often easy to just blame airbrushing, parents, peers, the media, advertisers and marketers for poor body image. But at some point, we must step back and take responsibility for our own actions. We must personally accept a degree of blame.

What? Why?

The decisions about which images and messages are to be presented in popular culture are not made by an evil, scheming individual living in an ivory tower on another planet.

Decisions are made by men and women in boardrooms around the world. Scattered around these boardrooms you're likely to find sales figures, projected profit forecasts, and a bunch of other information to show whether or not an advertisement, song, product, brand, logo, or program is working. If sales targets are met and if the magazine sells, these images or messages will continue to appear in popular culture – no matter how unrealistic or damaging they are to your body image.

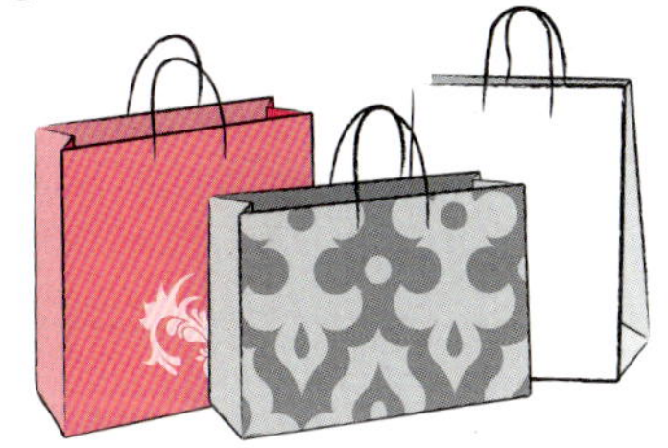

Now we can whine and complain all we want about ultra-skinny models and the lack of positive, healthy role models in popular culture… but we'll let you in on a secret: the decision-makers –

such as advertisers, magazine editors, and music industry executives - couldn't care less!

Their number one concern is a figure… but a numerical figure, not your figure in a swimsuit. Making you feel good about yourself is not their job…it's yours!

You might not agree with it but you can do something about it. Just keep this simple formula in mind:

Supply = Demand

Be a responsible consumer. Popular culture doesn't create itself. It follows demand. Like we said before, magazines feature celebrity diet tricks on the cover because you, or someone like you, buys those magazines.

The simple truth is:
we created popular culture.

But here's the good news: we also have the power to change popular culture. If you don't like the messages you're hearing, reading or seeing in popular culture, don't support the brand, the product, and the company with your hard-earned dollar. As a single consumer, you are more powerful than you can possibly imagine!

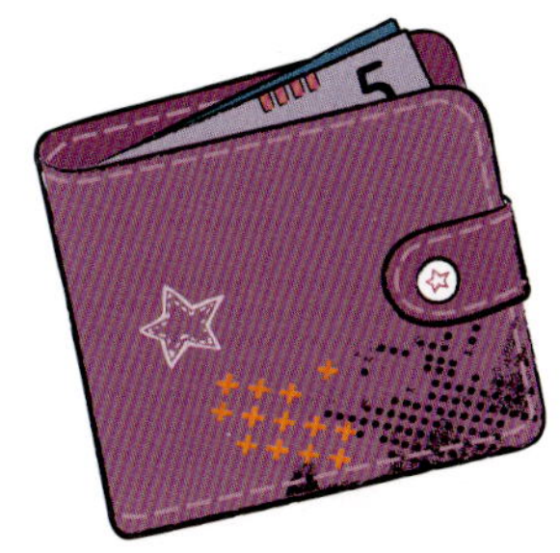

So now that you're armed with the knowledge to make media savvy decisions for yourself, don't be part of the problem. Be part of the solution! It's really a lot easier than you might think. You can send all the petition emails you want but nothing has a greater impact and reaches the decision makers faster than where your money goes.

So don't buy the magazine, do change the channel, close the website, and leave the product on the shelf. These days there are more and more great alternatives out there – like certain magazines featuring positive, healthy role models that won't deflate your self-esteem. So there's no excuse for fueling the distortion of body image with your spending habits.

Homework

- Think of ways that you can be a responsible consumer. Perhaps you could cancel that subscription to the magazine that makes you feel bad about yourself when you read it.

Chapter Seven

Give your body image a boost

By now we hope you've got a much better idea of how popular culture shapes your body image. You should also realise just how unrealistic media images really are. It's awesome if you're taking proactive steps with this new information and empowerment by changing your spending, viewing, reading, and listening habits. It feels great to have control over your body image instead of having it controlled by others!

Unfortunately, change doesn't happen overnight - especially when we're dealing with deeply ingrained human psychology. So let's be realistic. In the short term, advertising images will still be digitally altered to some extent. Anatomically 'perfect' males and females will still be used in music videos and body bullies will continue to reign the school yard. So what should you do about that? Well, you can start by reading Chapter One again - especially the bit about 'The benefits of positive body image'. But here are some more tips on how to develop a positive body image:

- Surround yourself with positive peers and colleagues who don't make you feel bad about yourself. Your environment should feel positive, be nurturing, uplifting and inspiring. It shouldn't be degrading or discouraging.
- Set realistic role models. Looking up to a digitally enhanced image is not a realistic role model. Role models should make you feel good about yourself and make you feel empowered. If your role model makes you feel inferior, then you are looking up to the wrong person.
- Don't judge yourself by physical features alone. Your weight will change but intelligence and academic achievements never do.
- Don't compare yourself with other people. Celebrate your individuality and embrace the things that make you unique and make you YOU!

Accept who you are, especially your flaws. You can do this by focusing on your great personality instead of that little pimple.

Remember that loving your body the way it is does not make you egotistical. It makes you smart and powerful in the most profound way. And there is nothing wrong with that!

Confidence is attractive. It's your best weapon. So go ahead and be proud of who you are!

We could write so much more on this but, truth be known, you probably have a bus to catch or an exam to study for so that's it for now.

So next time you pick up a magazine, watch a video clip, see a billboard or television ad, you'll be more media literate and have a better understanding of what goes on 'behind the scenes'. We hope that we've given you the knowledge and skills to navigate the popular culture maze with your body image and self-esteem intact.

Homework

- Think about what makes you beautiful or attractive. Except, your answers can't be physical (such as a 'skinny waist' or 'big muscles') and it can't be something you buy (like clothes or jewellery). For example, confidence and honesty make you beautiful – but they aren't physical and can't be bought.

But, wait, there is still one other question we need to address:

Does my bum look big in this ad?

The answer?

Who cares!!!

About the author
Lisa Cox

BA Business (Communications)
BA Arts (Media)

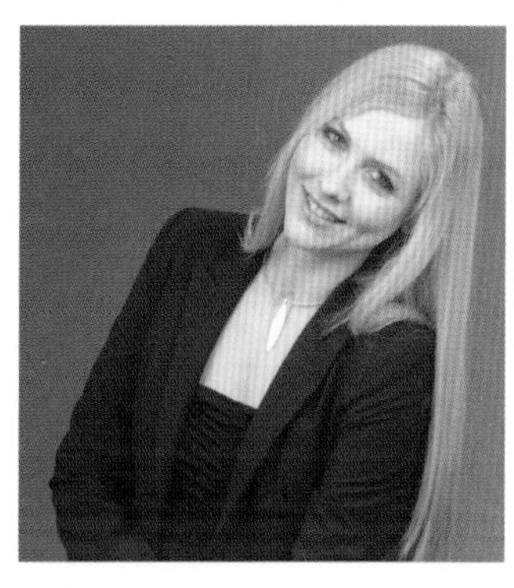

Lisa Cox spent nearly a decade studying and working in the media and advertising industry. She also spent time working as a fashion model so, has seen the distortion and manipulation of body image in popular culture from both sides of the camera lens.

Described as "an advocate for healthy body image" (The Sunday Mail) and the "body image spokeswoman" (Mindfood Magazine), Lisa now shares her insight with youth to promote media literacy and positive body image.

Acknowledgements

We wish to acknowledge and sincerely thank the following people for their valued input and feedback towards this book:

Amanda Dunne
Art Director and Media Consultant

Linnie Sharma
Berlin based Writer, Media Commentator and body image Consultant
www.dreyecandy.com

Sophee McPhee
Editor, UP! Magazine
www.upmagazine.com.au

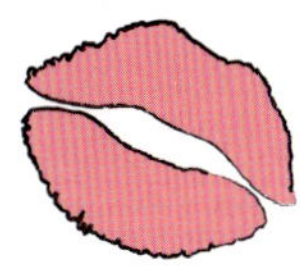

Peggy Kubat-Szucs Executive Director
Me Without Measure Foundation – An eating disorder organisation
www.mewithoutmeasure.org

Tracey Cox
Advertising Account Manager

Renee Kelly
Childhood Psychologist